Paleo Diet for Beginners
Lose Weight and Start Living the Paleo Lifestyle. Easy Paleo Diet Recipes for Weight Loss.

JANE JOHNSON

Copyright © 2015 Jane Johnson

All rights reserved.

ISBN: 1517098246
ISBN-13: 978-1517098247

CONTENTS

Introduction i

Chapter 1 – The Paleo Foundation 1

    Why Grains Can Cause Weight and Health Problems 4

    Why Sugar Can Cause Weight and Health Problems 6

Chapter 2 – The Paleo Diet Guidelines 9

    List of No-No's 14

    Eat When You Are Hungry 15

    Stress and Eating 16

Chapter 3 – Paleo Diet Recipes 18

    Zucchini and Eggs 19

    Fruit and Nut Spinach Salad 20

    Eggplant Dip 21

    Lamb Kabobs 22

    Lemon-Pepper Tilapia 24

    Rosemary Chicken Breast Salad 25

    Oven Stew 26

    Fruit Mix Salad 27

Conclusion 28

Introduction

For the last several years, there seems to have been more diet trends that have come and gone and the established groups have remained consistent (Weight Watchers, Jenny Craig, etc.). In those years, one diet thought to be a trend has proven it has staying power: the Paleo Diet. The reason: it works, especially for weight loss. In fact, studies have shown that when combined with exercise, the Paleo diet helps you lose more pounds than the others.

An incredibly simple and common sense diet, the Paleo diet is based on the types of foods anthropologists and others have proven that early humans consumed. Fresh fish, meat, vegetables, fruits, nuts and seeds are the foundation. It excludes dairy, grains and processed foods to the benefit of your waistline and your health.

Where did they ever come up with it you may ask? Well, it actually has its roots in the 1970s, when a doctor and scholar named Walter Voetglin surmised that Western society needed to wake up and could be much healthier if everyone returned to the basics that the earliest human ancestors ate.

He pinpointed the Paleolithic era, about 11,000 years ago, a pre-agricultural time when humans were hunter-gatherers, living off the land. A time before excessive processing of our foods and well before GMOs.

As society became ever-more industrialized and more and more people became urbanites, the diet of the average Westerner was becoming more dependent on processed and packaged foods—and sugar. Believing something had to be done if the population was to have a bright future, free of obesity and rampant diabetes (to name just two of the illnesses that were on the rise), Dr. Voetglin came up with the foundation for today's Paleo diet.

It didn't really take hold in the Western world until the publication of *The Paleo Diet*, by Loren Collins, in 2002. Providing people with what seemed an easier and scientifically sound principle for losing weight and feeling better, the book took off, especially with celebrities expounding the Paleo diet's virtues and sports figures attributing it with their better performance.

Very recently (2015), there have been various articles suggesting that our "cavemen" ancestors did not necessarily eat the way Dr. Voetglin and Collins had written and that there is obviously no "one" Paleo diet because different regions provided different natural resources—a land-locked village, for example, would not have had access to an abundance of fish, one of the staples of Collins' Paleo diet.

As well, there is evidence that Paleolithic peoples ate grains, starch and other carbohydrates as a regular part of their nutrition, all of which are "no-no's" on the Paleo diet. The academics are making too literal a case of the reference to "Paleo" in my estimation. Of course we are not trying to eat *exactly* as they did. But we are trying to eat cleaner and with more mind to the nutritive value of our foods.

No matter the history, the academic principles the Paleo diet is built on will be debated in scholarly circles for years, I am sure. What cannot be argued though is that the Paleo diet works, especially when it comes to weight loss.

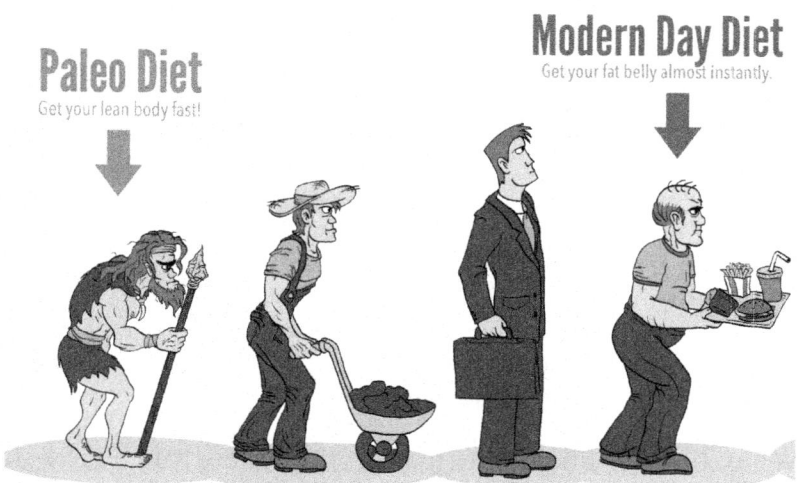

It comes down to the Paleo diet being based on sound nutritional principles. We all know we need to avoid added and hidden sugars, chemicals, bad fats, and processed foods. Even recognized experts do not deny the helpfulness of the Paleo diet's promotion of avoiding high-glycemic foods (those that raise blood glucose sugar levels) and eliminating inflammation-causing fats (such as those found in fast foods and deep fried foods).

One of the other (and some would say best) elements of the Paleo diet is how easy it is. I mean incredibly simple to follow and actually enjoy. There is no calorie-counting, no little cards to carry to every restaurant and no weekly group weigh-ins. There is no obsessing over how many grams of a particular nutrient is in your morning meal.

In fact, following diets that only track calories actually can detract from a weight loss goal because 400 calories of potato chips does not affect your body in the same way 400 calories of fresh apple slices would. It just makes sense when viewed from that perspective.

What does it all mean in the end? Well, the Paleo diet of today is essentially a healthy and well-thought out interpretation of what made our earliest ancestors healthier than we are today. It means a return to cleaner, more nutrient-dense eating and, in the end, making simple, sensible choices.

> Anyone can do it and should if they want to live longer, healthier and more productive lives..

Chapter 1 – The Paleo Foundation

Proven to help weight loss (studies again have shown the Paleo diet coupled with exercise actually produces better weight-loss results long-term than many of the other diets on the market today), to ensure you have the building blocks for muscle and be in the best health of your life, Paleo eating is the ultimate in "basic" diets. In coordination with regular exercise, it has helped tens of thousands of people reach their potential.

The foundation is simple as well—our bodies have not really evolved or changed substantially since the Paleolithic era. Though the way we live our lives and how we get our food has changed drastically, of course, with food processing techniques and advances in agriculture evolving exponentially, our essential body chemistry and our internal systems that allow us to digest and use food as fuel have not changed with them.

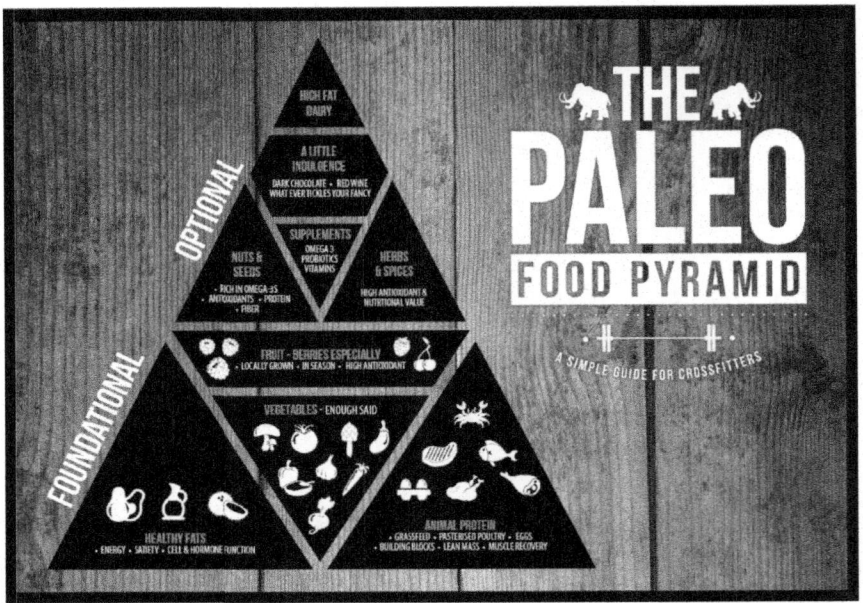

The average human in the Paleolithic era had the same internal organs and they worked as ours do. So why were they generally more muscular and less overweight than us? Why did they suffer less from the diseases that we do, like diabetes, heart diseases, etc.?

Part of it has to do with lifestyle of course. They didn't have any of the modern conveniences we do today and of course they literally fought to put food on their tables. However, Dr. Voetglin also attributed this to *what* they put on their tables and subsequently in their bodies.

With the advent of agriculture, early Paleolithic man went from being hunter-gatherers—always on the move whether it be tracking and catching the animals they used for meat or out in the fields and forests gathering roots and berries to supplement their stores of food—to settled in one place, planting and harvesting and keeping animals in herds.

Fast forward a few millennia and you have the grain and sugar dependent diet of modern North America. Combined with how static and immobile our lifestyle is—you do not even have to leave the house to get groceries in many cities; one click and they are delivered to your door—and we have the perfect environment for the explosion of obesity and illnesses today.

Why Grains Can Cause Weight and Health Problems

When we talk about grains, we are talking about everything from your cereal to breads. Anything made with wheat, rye, etc. The problem with grains is that they are made up of carbohydrates and too many carbohydrates causes issues in your blood sugar. From there it compounds and causes weight gain.

The science of it, simplistically is your body can only convert so many carbs to sugar that can be used for energy for on a cellular level. Too many carbs means too much sugar and that raises your blood sugar levels (the Glycemic Index). The body then releases insulin to control the blood sugars to manageable level.

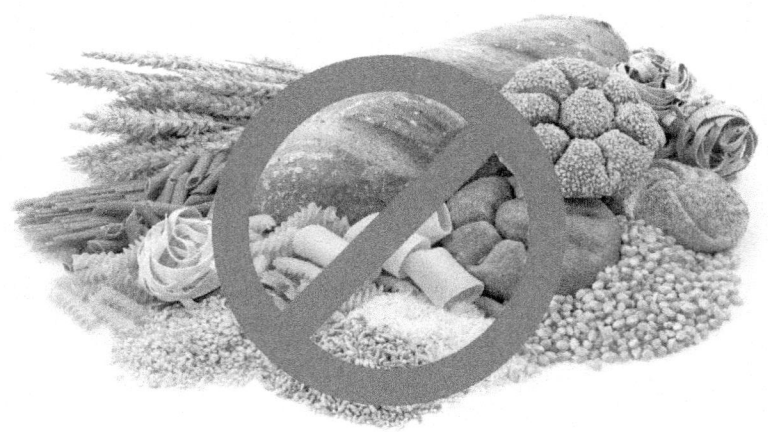

What it cannot control it has to store in fat cells.

Cells can become resistant to the effects of the insulin over time and stop doing what they are supposed to do, meaning let the insulin bring the sugars down. So your body combats that by producing more insulin driving the sugars into the fat cells. Type II Diabetes, weight gain and the like follow.

Another specific trait of most grains is that they contain gluten and lectins. Gluten is a protein found in grains such as rye, wheat and barley. Intolerance to gluten is responsible for a whole host of chronic conditions, such as dermatitis, joint pain, reproductive issues, acid reflux and the like.

Lectins are naturally occurring but are toxins in grains meant to protect the plant from being eaten. Ironic isn't it? Literally the lectins are geared to stopping us from consuming the grain. Not lethal, though, the toxins do play havoc with a person's gastrointestinal tract, preventing it from repairing itself from normal wear and tear. As with gluten intolerance, lectins are responsible for an array of GI issues plaguing modern society (Irritable Bowel Syndrome is one).

Why Sugar Can Cause Weight and Health Problems

Sugar has become so prevalent in our culture that it is in even our savory foods. Addiction to sugar is in the eyes of some an epidemic. Though our bodies need sugar (to burn off calories and provide energy for our cells), we are overlooking our bodies to the point that those cells are crying for help in processing the overload.

Diabetes, inflammatory diseases, even acne, plague our lives and keep getting worse with each generation. The Paleo diet eliminates all sugar except that which naturally occurs in the fresh fruits and vegetables eaten.

Why? Well sugar is a complicated little crystal. On the one hand, it is a simple carbohydrate (what all other carbohydrates are converted into in the cells), necessary for your body to create energy to survive. You need it to survive.

Where the problems begin is when we consume added sugar or artificial sugars. It is not necessary to include sugary foods in your diet if you are getting it from natural sources. And remember grains? Well, as mentioned, they are eliminated in the Paleo diet partly because they are carbs and carbs convert to sugars, adding to the amount you are taking in.

Too much sugar can cause inflammation throughout the body, not just in the joints. It is the body's over-reaction of the immune system fighting what it perceives to be threats. It can cause what are called "spikes" in your blood sugar levels creating the spiral described earlier.

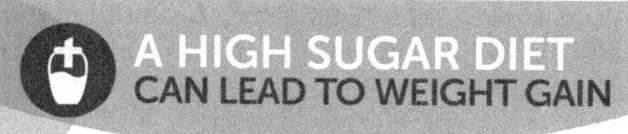

A high sugar diet can lead to weight gain, which increases your risk of cancer

OVERWEIGHT AND OBESITY COULD CAUSE 10 TYPES OF CANCER

1 IN 20
UK CANCERS ARE LINKED TO WEIGHT

Oesophagus

Breast
after menopause

Liver

Pancreas

Kidney

Bowel

Womb

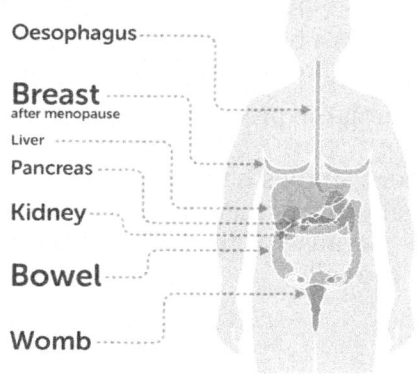

Being overweight may also cause gallbladder, aggressive prostate and ovarian cancer

WE WILL **BEAT** CANCER SOONER
cruk.org

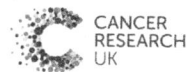
CANCER RESEARCH UK

Besides this, foods with a high sugar content contain a high calorie content and if those calories are not burned off they are stored as fat. On top of that, the empty calories can contribute to nutrient deficiencies and will most definitely cause cavities, Sugar provides an easily digestible energy source for the bad bacteria in your mouth.

Sugar is broken down into two simple sugars before it enters your bloodstream from your digestive tract: glucose and fructose. Glucose is found in every living cell on the planet but it is not necessary in your diet. If we do not get it in our diets, our bodies can produce it.

Fructose has no redeeming value though and does harm in large quantities as it is stored in your liver if your system is overloaded with it. A little bit, say from a piece of fruit, will be turned into glycogen and stored for future use.

But if the liver is already "full" to capacity with glycogen, eating more sugar overloads it and it is forced to convert the fructose to fat within the liver. This leads to a "fatty liver". A condition most often associated with alcoholics, fatty liver is on the rise because of our "sweet" Western lifestyle.

Cutting out sugar for the Paleo diet has another important health benefit: it can help lower your cholesterol. For decades now, it was always thought that "bad" or saturated fats were the cause of high cholesterol, the precursor to heart disease.

Recent studies have proved that is a misconception and that it is actually sugar that is one of the major leading drivers of heart disease because of the harmful effects of fructose on metabolism within the cells.

Chapter 2 – The Paleo Diet Guidelines

To ensure you get the most out of the Paleo diet, there are a number of guidelines you can follow. And remember before you start any diet or exercise regime, check with your doctor that it is safe for you to do so.

Your first step is going to be to clean out your cupboards, pantry and refrigerator. Donate to the food bank or find a friend who would appreciate the food if you can. Or perhaps to be frugal, try to finish up what is there now before you go for groceries and then you can shop with Paleo in mind.

You are going to be eliminating the sugary treats, the processed, pre-packaged dinners, the soda—you no longer want them or need them. You are going to be cleaning up your diet.

Next, make your grocery list based on the following foundation of foods:

1. Meats: beef, chicken, pork, etc.
2. Fish and seafood: salmon, trout, haddock, shrimp, shellfish, etc.
3. Eggs

4. Vegetables: broccoli, kale, peppers, onions, carrots, tomatoes, etc.
5. Fruits: apples, oranges, bananas, etc.
6. Nuts and seeds: almonds, walnuts, etc.
7. Healthy fats and oils: butter, coconut oil, olive oil, etc.

When shopping for anything from the above list, it is important to try to buy the freshest, most natural of the choices offered. This means organic pasture-raised beef or local pesticide-free apples and the like. The more organic the better. Now you may also be concerned about your carbon footprint so shop to that guideline if you want to.

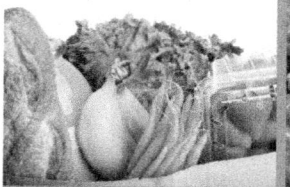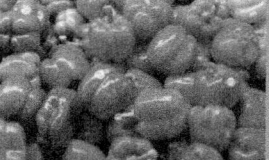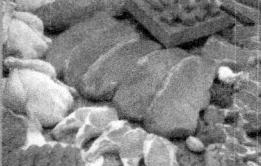

SHOPPING LIST

Pecan Pie Butter with Apples
Servings: Makes 2 cups.
- 1/2 cup raw almonds
- 1 1/2 cup raw pecans
- 2 pitted dates (we used medjool)
- 2 tsp salt
- 1/2 orange, zested
- 1/4 cup almond oil (might take a little more) a few tart apples, my favorite is Pink Lady dried cranberries or dark chocolate chips

Jerky
Servings: Makes 1 batch.
- 2 lbs ribeye, trimmed of the big hunks of fat
- pineapple core & rinds
- cilantro stems
- ginger peel
- sweetener of choice
- water
- 3 TB coconut aminos

Tuna Stuffed Avocado
Servings: Makes 6 to 8 servings.
- 3-4 ripe avocados
- 4 cans of Trader Joe's tuna packed in water
- 3 green onions
- 3 celery stalks
- 1 palm full of dried dill
- 1 TB garlic powder
- fresh ground black pepper to taste
- grape tomatoes halved
- Ingredients to make 1 cup of Olive Oil Mayo:
- 1 egg
- 1 1/2 TB apple cider vinegar
- pinch of sea salt
- few shakes of cayenne pepper
- 1 tsp yellow mustard
- 1 cup olive oil
- 1/2 cup raw almonds
- 1 1/2 cup raw pecans
- 2 pitted dates (we used medjool)
- 2 tsp salt
- 1/2 orange, zested
- 1/4 cup almond oil (might take a little more) a few tart apples, my favorite is Pink Lady dried cranberries or dark chocolate chips

Smoked Salmon Nori Roll
Servings: Makes 1 roll.
- cucumber, sliced lengthwise into flat strips
- vegetables of choice: celery, red pepper, and/or carrot sticks
- tahini
- smoked salmon
- nori sheets

Taro Chips
Servings: Makes 1 batch.
- taro root, peeled
- duck fat, lard, or coconut oil
- salt to taste

Rutabaga and Onion Hash Browns
Servings: Makes 1 to 2 servings.
- 5 oz. peeled and diced rutabaga, 1/2" dice or smaller (about 1 cup)
- 2 oz. chopped onion (1/4 cup)
- 1 TB traditional fat of choice
- dash each of salt and black pepper
- sausage or any cooked leftover meat

Breakfast Squash and Sausage
Servings: Makes 2 to 4 servings.
- 2 delicata squash, cut in half and deseeded
- 1 TB coconut oil
- 1 tsp ground cinnamon
- 1/2 tsp sea salt
- 6oz ground pork breakfast sausage (you can use any ground meat you like, just make sure it's flavorful)
- 4 eggs, whisked
- ground fennel and fennel fronds, for garnish (optional)

It may take some getting used to, but your diet should also be high in fat, moderate in animal protein and low to moderate in carbohydrates. (I know I said no carbs but you'll see what I mean shortly.)

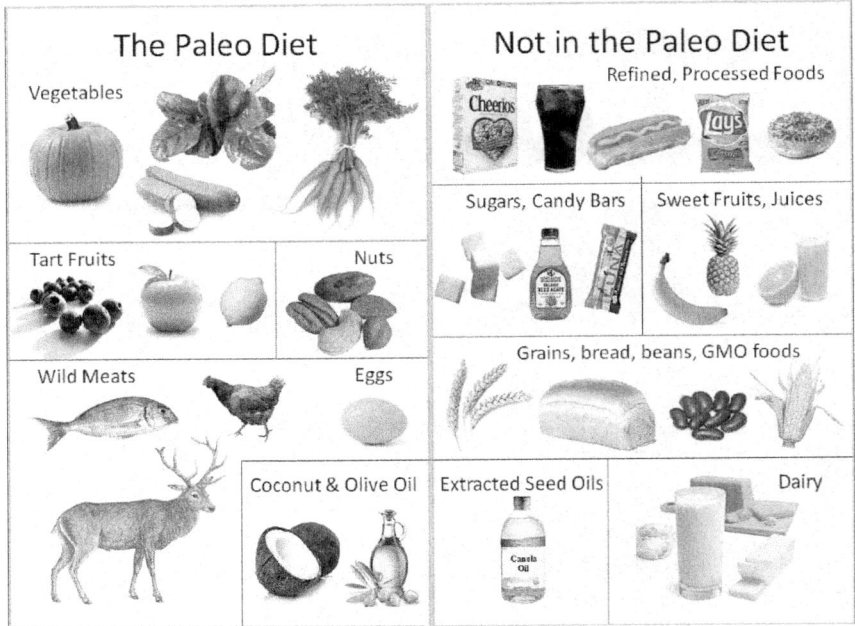

Another thing that will differ perhaps is there is no calorie-counting nor portion-control, as with anything, eat in moderation. Listen to your body. When it signals you are full, put the utensil down.

When it comes to fats, do not be afraid to eat generous amounts—coconut oil and butter are good examples of the fats that will give your body the right fuel. Just be sure they are from high-quality sources.

Portions are loosely guided by the particular food group. Good amounts of animal protein should be consumed. Fatty cuts are fine and every meal that includes this kind of protein needs to include a fat. Another good practice is to use the bones to make stocks and broths for recipes.

Fresh or frozen vegetables can be served in generous portions. Cooked or raw, it does not matter, just once again ensure you serve them with some kind of fat. And this is where you can make up for the loss of grains and their fiber content. Use sweet potatoes to provide not only the fiber but also a good source of non-toxic carbs.

Fruits and nuts should be on the smaller scale portion-wise. You also need to look for those that provide the lowest sugar content but are also high in anti-oxidants. When it comes to the type of nuts you choose, look for those rich in omega-3, low in omerga-6 and low in polyunsaturated fats (macadamia nuts fit this bill). Please note: If you have an auto-immune disease, digestive problems or want to speed up weight-loss, eliminate this category of food.

Choosing animal protein should be guided by the "purer the better". Beef from cattle allowed to graze in a pesticide-free pasture or eggs from free-range chickens are worth the cost. If it is impossible for you to buy these types, whether it is availability issues or your limited budget, just make sure you look for lean cuts of meat or Omega-3 enriched eggs and supplement the lost "good fat" source with coconut oil or butter.

List of No-No's

As you already have read, grains should no longer be part of your meal plans. This means no breads, rolls, cereals, pastries, and so on. As well, legumes such as kidney beans, black-eyed peas, soy and peanuts are not on the menu.

Cut out any hydrogenated or even partially hydrogenated and vegetable oils. This means no sunflower, corn or vegetable oils or margarine, to name a few. Olive or avocado oils are good for you but do not cook with them (it has to do with how they break down under high heat). Just employ them as drizzles or dressings.

Added sugar of any kind has to go. So do not buy any sodas, juice boxes, frozen concentrate, and those are only the most obvious sources. Check labels for sugar content. And stay away from packaged cookies, bars, etc. The rule of thumb is if it is packaged in a box, leave it on the shelf.

Dairy other than butter (and perhaps heavy cream) is not a part of the Paleo diet, but if you find you cannot live without it, consider buying only raw, full fat or fermented products.

Eat When You Are Hungry

What? Say that again. "Eat when you are hungry." I bet not too many diets you have been on made that a rule.

One of the most common sense rules if you can call it that, this belief of the Paleo diet is based on the idea that you need to listen to your body. This also of course applies to stopping eating when your body says it is full. Many people struggling with their weight have actually put their systems so out of sync by overloading them with sugar that they have disrupted the satiety center of their brains. That means that they do not ever feel sated or full.

This part will get easier with the elimination of sugars. You will be allowing your brain to let you know when you are truly hungry and it will know when you are full. And if you skip a meal or two, which happens in everyone's hectic lives, do not worry. Unlike other plans, the Paleo diet does not revolve around six small meals a day or three big ones. It is about the natural pace of your body.

Stress and Eating

By now, you know the various ways stress has a negative effect on our lives. It is probably a topic of at least one news show a day wherever you are from. It is hard to say if we have "more" stress than Paleolithic people did—running from a ferocious hungry carnivore with only a spear for defence would be pretty stressful I think—but we do have different stresses and they are coming at us in a more constant stream than ever before.

Like any other wellness program, the Paleo diet will work best if you eliminate as many stresses from your life as you can. So maybe give in and let your child take the bus to school. You can give yourself a few minutes alone to be ready for the day at work. Or try out a yoga class at the local recreation center. Many of them let you pay as you go and some even offer a free class to try it out. Yoga in particular provides you with both exercise and meditation as well as being a gentler introduction to activity if you have not been exercising for a while. Little things do help.

And get a good night's sleep, the eight hours your mother told you to all those years ago. This means preparing for bed properly: turn off the TV, iPad, laptop and smartphone at least an hour before you crawl under the sheets. Another tip is to try to make bedtime a consistent time each night (or day if you work shift work). Maybe even buy some new high quality sheets as a treat. It may be the incentive you need to fall off to sleep more quickly.

To assist nutritionally, you may want to consider adding a couple of supplements to your diet now. Vitamin D and probiotics are suggested to complement the Paleo diet. You should also think about getting your magnesium, iodine and

Vitamin K levels checked. Again, consult with your doctor before you start taking any kind of supplements.

Chapter 3 – Paleo Diet Recipes

Now for the fun stuff: making the meals. Remember, you can always adapt your favorite recipes to the Paleo diet by finding substitutes that fit the eating plan. Almond flour can be used in place of wheat flour to make a quick and easy microwave bread. Chopped carrots can be used in place of white sugar in your favorite spaghetti sauce recipes. It is all about trial and error.

The following are just a handful of recipes that incorporate the Paleo diet ingredients. I hope they will appeal, but you know you can also experiment with your own. Remember there is not just one form of "Paleo". It can be guided by regional availability and personal traditions.

Zucchini and Eggs

Start your day off right with this unusual and yummy combination.

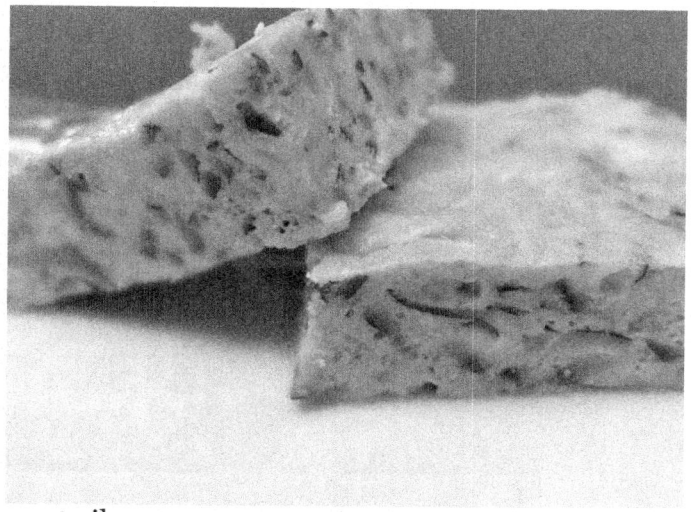

2 tsp coconut oil

1 small zucchini, sliced thinly

1 egg, beaten

Salt and pepper to taste

Heat a small skillet over medium heat. Pour in oil and sauté the zucchini until just tender. Spread the zucchini in an even layer and pour beaten egg over the top, covering it. Cook egg until firm and season with salt and pepper to taste.

Fruit and Nut Spinach Salad

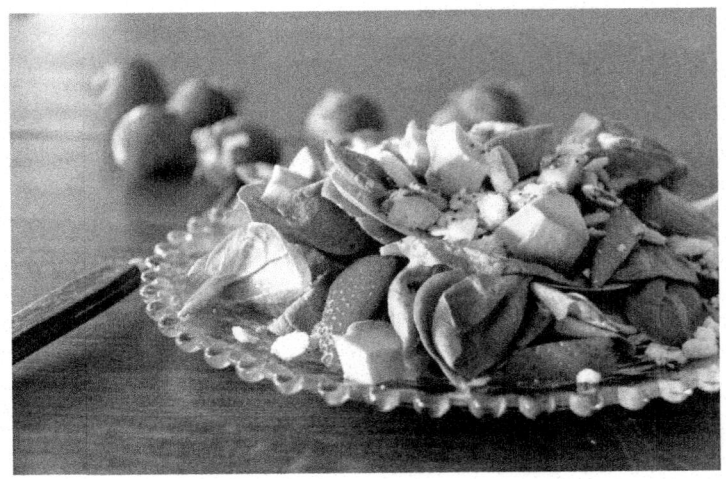

Combining a number of Paleo elements, this is a delicious side dish or a great midday lunch.

2 to 3 oz baby spinach

1 navel orange, peeled and cut into small pieces

1 Empire apple, peeled and cut into small pieces

Large handful of walnut halves

½ c chopped red onion

In bowl, combine ingredients; toss with your favorite oil and vinegar dressing.

Eggplant Dip

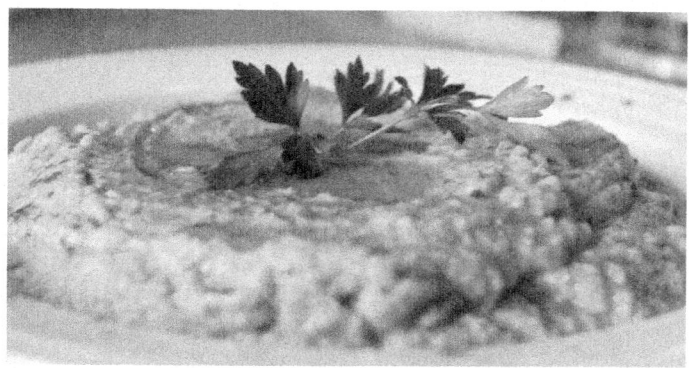

Entertaining can even incorporate Paleo.

1 large eggplant

1 clove of garlic

¼ c extra-virgin olive oil

2 tbsp lemon juice

½ tsp salt

Pinch of cayenne pepper

Pinch of paprika

Cut four evenly spaced 1-inch deep slits lengthwise into the eggplant; place with garlic on baking sheet and roast on 450 degrees until garlic is soft and eggplant is browned and fork tender. Peel the eggplant and remove and large seed clusters. Transfer to a medium-sized mixing bowl. Squeeze the individual garlic buds from the clove in with the eggplant and with a fork, mash well. Whisk in oil, lemon juice and cayenne. Serve as a dip for veggies.

Lamb Kabobs

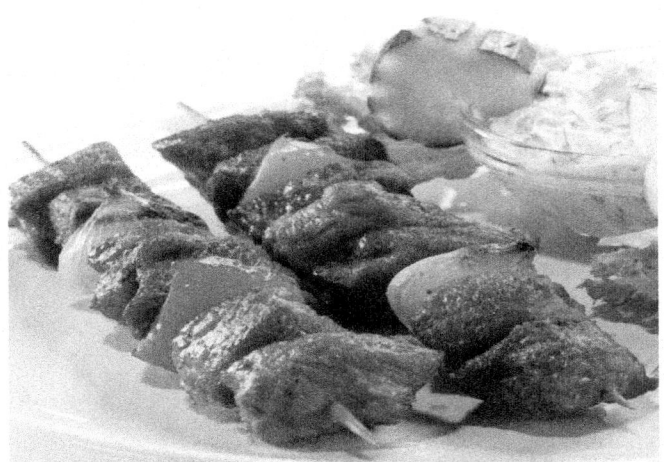

An alternative to the red meat that Paleo is famous for.

½ c of raw cashew nuts or blanched almonds

6 green hot peppers, seeded and chopped

½ onion, chopped

2 tbsp chopped ginger root

2 tbsp butter, melted

1 egg

1 egg yolk

1 ¾ tsp salt

1 tsp turmeric

½ tsp white pepper

¼ tsp cayenne

¼ tsp each ground cardamom, cinnamon, ground cloves, ground cumin, nutmeg and black pepper

1 ½ kb ground lamb

1/3 c finely chopped coriander

In food processor, whir together cashew nuts, peppers, onion, ginger root and butter until a smooth paste. In a large bowl, whisk egg with extra yolk; whisk in cashew mixture and all other ground spices until thoroughly mixed. Add lamb and coriander and with oiled hands or a wooden spoon, mix thoroughly. Refrigerate for at least 2 hours (to a maximum of 24). With moistened hands, form 16 balls, using ¼ cup of the lamb mixture for each. Shape each into 4 inch long sausage shape and put on skewers. Grill until no longer pink in center (on a barbeque, about 10 minutes).

Lemon-Pepper Tilapia

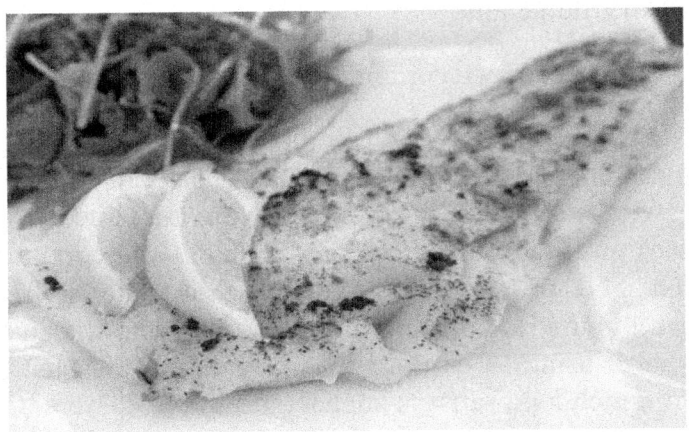

One of the more popular types of fish, this is an easy recipe to whip up when you do not have much time.

¼ c almond flour

½ tsp lemon-pepper seasoning

2 firm tilapia fillets

1 tsp unsalted butter

Mix together the flour and lemon-pepper seasoning, then dip each fish fillet in the flour mixture. Ina hot frying pan, melt the butter. Drop in fish and cook for about four minutes per side or until slightly brown. Serve immediately.

Rosemary Chicken Breast Salad

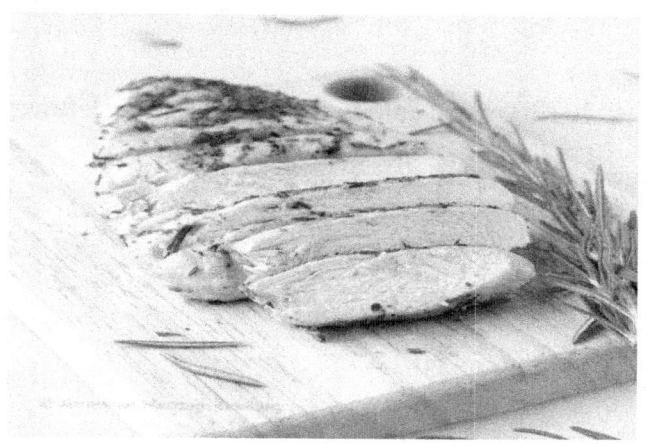

Marinade:

1 tbsp chopped fresh rosemary or 2 tsp crumbled dry oregano

1 tbsp extra-virgin olive oil

½ tsp each of salt and pepper

Suggested Salad Greens

6 c Italian lettuce mix (such as escarole, curly endive and romaine)

1 c halved cherry tomatoes

In bowl, whisk marinade ingredients. Add chicken and roll to coat. Marinate for at least 30 minutes or, refrigerated, for up to 24 hours. Grill chicken over medium-high heat, turning once. When no longer pink in the thickest part, remove from heat and slice in thin strips. Serve over salad and dress with your favorite dressing.

Oven Stew

A hearty dish to serve on a cold night (and great for leftovers).

2 ¼ lbs stew beef, cut bite size or larger

2 medium onions, cut into quarters

5 medium potatoes, quartered

5 medium carrots, chopped

2 celery stocks, sliced

28 oz stewed tomatoes (if not homemade, ensure there is no sugar added)

2 c beef stock (preferably homemade)

1 tsp lemon juice

½ tsp salt

1 tsp pepper

Put the first five ingredients in a medium sized roaster. Mix the remaining ingredients together in a bowl. Pour over the contents of the roaster and cover. Bake in 400 degree over for four hours until tender.

Fruit Mix Salad

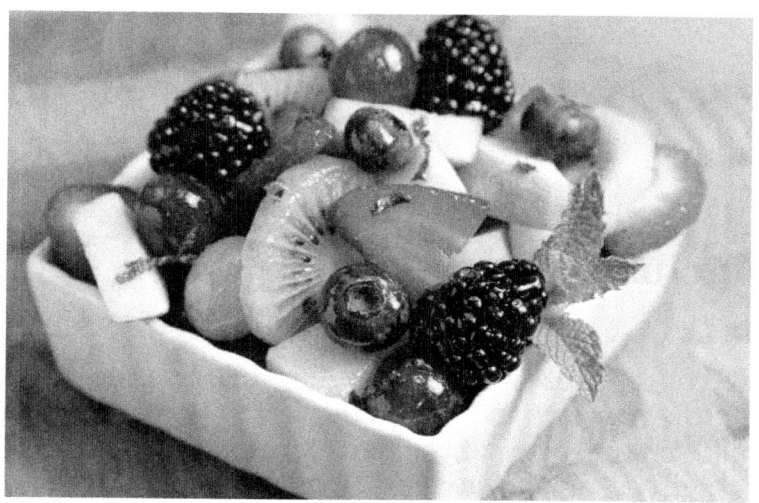

Because we all crave something sweet, this should satisfy your sweet tooth.

2 oranges, peeled and chopped

1 c seedless red grapes

½ c pitted and halved Bing cherries

¼ c golden raisins

¼ c pitted and chopped dates

¼ c walnut halves

Combine all the ingredients in a large salad bowl and toss gently to combine. Leave to allow the juices to mingle and create a natural dressing.

Conclusion

Now you are ready to start feeling better and lose weight using the pointers and tips in this book. Remember that you should always okay any dietary changes with your doctor before proceeding. But chances are he or she will be thrilled simply that you are taking control of your health and eliminating sugar.

From getting rid of sugar to eating when you are hungry, it is a relatively simple diet to follow. In just a few days it won't even feel like you are on a diet. And the energy, slimmer waistline and better skin will keep you eating like a "caveman" for the rest of your life, I am sure.

Remember: it is all about eating simply, more naturally. So read those labels (sugar lurks everywhere) and try to buy organic, grass-fed, free-range and so on. You will be surprised at what you have been missing out on just in the taste of this kind of food.

It is a way back to basic diet but it is wonderfully satisfying and should actually serve to curb cravings you thought would never stop. As discussed, sugar creates cravings for sugar. Without it the body will balance and all you will have to do is break the psychological habit.

And you will not miss sugary drinks and chocolate bars. But if you do, any good dieter knows that a cheat now and then is not the end of the world. In fact it might ensure you do not just toss in the towel and give up.

When it comes to recipes, try to find ways to substitute the Paleo diet ingredients for the usual. You can even make an unleavened bread if you use a nut flour like almond. There are so many options, all you have to do is a little research.

Remember to rewrite your grocery list with Paleo in mind. And a tip for grocery shopping that has come to public notice in the past few years is to shop the outside of the grocery store. The "bad stuff" is in the center aisles.

If you take notice next time you are in your local grocery store you will see that all of the "fresh" food is indeed on the outer part of the store, from the meats to the vegetables. So stick to those departments and you will easily fill your cart with Paleo diet staples.

Isn't it nice to know the Paleo diet is not really eating like a caveman? It is not just red meat and root vegetables. It is a nutritionally sound option for anyone who is suffering with many of today's most prevalent illnesses and it is a tasty and intelligent way to go about weight loss.

Once you have been on the diet for a month, you should have increased energy. So that would be the perfect time to introduce a new fitness class, perhaps. Or if you do not enjoy class settings, try a web-based yoga class. Any kind of movement and exercise is going to speed up your weight loss.

One more thing. Do not forget to not just east right. You also need to use the tips given in the book about getting a good night's sleep and taking time to declutter your life and lessen you stress. Take up a hobby, read a book, or go for a walk.

At least the Paleo diet will not add to the stress. Based on easy to access real foods and simple enough for even a child to enjoy, the Paleo diet will soon be so easy you will be wondering why you did not do it sooner.

Thank you for reading. I hope you enjoy it. You can leave your honest feedback.